INTERMITTENT FASTING

DIET PLAN

the complete guide to Healthy Life Style and Extreme Weight loss to Master the Secrets of Fasting and to Promote Longevity.

6 BOOK OF 12

"Update chapter 4 second edition "

By Melissa White

3

Chapter 1. Intermittent Fasting's Role in Cancer Initiation, Progression, and Metastasis

The job of dietary limitation regimens like caloric limitation, ketogenic diet and intermittent fasting being developed of tumors has been distinguished through bountiful preclinical examinations. In any case, the ends are questionable. We intend to audit the important creature concentrates deliberately and give help to additional clinical investigations.

Written works on relationship between dietary limitation and malignancy distributed in ongoing twenty years were extensively looked. Creature model, tumor type, taking care of routine, study length, test size, significant result, end, quality appraisal score and the interferential step of malignant growth were separated from each qualified examination. We broke down the tumor occurrence rates from 21 examinations about caloric limitation.

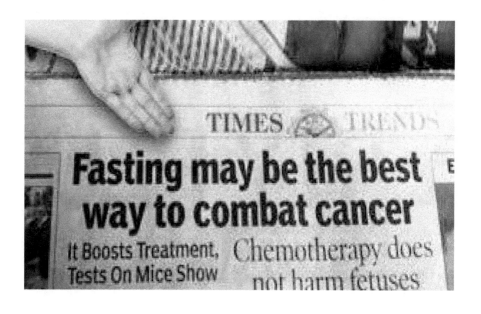

1.1 Introduction

Malignancy was the subsequent driving reason for mortality worldwide and its rate has been expanding during the most recent many years. Epidemiological investigations report that diet assumes a significant part in the commencement, advancement and movement of basic diseases. For quite a long time, dietary limitation has been generally perceived with medical advantages and reliably been appeared to broaden life expectancy in different warm blooded subjects. Its anticancer impacts have as of late been recognized through various creature tests. Among different dietary limitation regimens, caloric limitation (CR), intermittent fasting (IF) and starch limitation/ketogenic diet (KD) are the most examined strategies that are advantageous for malignancy counteraction.

CR forestalls tumorigenesis by diminishing metabolic rate and oxidative harm. The instrument behind intermittent fasting IF is generally straightforward: it defers tumor development by starving tumors from glucose for a brief period. KD used to treat obstinate seizures in youngsters for quite a long time is an eating routine made out of low carbs (typically under 50 g/day), high fat and enough proteins. KD can confine glucose for ATP creation and energy deduction in disease cells.

The current outcomes essentially start from creature models, like unconstrained model, compound incited model, transgenic model and relocated model. Since human clinical preliminaries of dietary limitation are amazingly uncommon, it is earnest to survey the current

9

accomplishments in regards to the malignancy preventive adequacy of dietary limitation in creature models. The present orderly audit was directed to examine the discoveries from the most important and ongoing investigations concerning the impacts of dietary limitation regimens on malignant growth counteraction.

1.2 Research and Inclusion Criteria

The consideration rules are: 1. concentrates on the anticancer impacts of CR, IF or KD; 2. considers utilizing creature models; 3. examines revealing in any event one of the result measures related with antitumor impacts. Studies in vitro and on human members were barred. Rehashed examines performed by a similar creator would not be incorporated.

The titles and edited compositions of the got articles were checked on by two commentators autonomously. Subsequent to barring the articles not gathering the incorporation standards, the two commentators read the entire entry of the leftover articles to ensure they genuinely met the consideration rules. Any contention was settled by conversation with the third commentator to arrive at agreement among all analysts.

Two analysts autonomously evaluated each included article as per a basic agenda of the Stroke Therapy Academic Industry Roundtable. The central issues of this agenda include: 1. performing suitable example size estimations; 2. characterizing consideration/rejection models deduced; 3. detailing the age of stochastic succession; 4. giving the technique for hiding intermittent allotment grouping; 5. detailing the explanations behind barring creatures from the last information examination; 6. wiping out result evaluation inclination; 7. announcing significant irreconcilable circumstances.

Two commentators autonomously separated information. Data including creature model, tumor type, taking care of routine, study length, test size, significant result, end, quality evaluation score and the interferential step of malignancy was separated from each investigation utilizing a preset structure.

Fifty nine examinations were associated with our framework audit. The elaborate investigations investigated parts of dietary limitation during inception, movement and metastasis of malignancy. About 90.9% of the significant investigations showed that caloric limitation plays an enemy of malignant growth job. Ketogenic diet was additionally emphatically connected with malignancy, which was shown by eight of the nine examinations. In any case, 37.5% of the connected examinations acquired an adverse end that intermittent fasting was not altogether preventive against malignant growth.

Eligible studies

The progression of search system is appeared. An aggregate of 1463 articles were distinguished and 1306 examinations were avoided subsequent to checking on title and theoretical, with a determination of 157 investigations for definite survey. 23 audits, ten cell examinations, and eight clinical preliminaries were thusly prohibited after full-text perusing as per the incorporation measures. Three rehashed distributed creature studies, and eight rehashed examines performed by a similar creator were avoided. Fifteen malignancy unimportant examinations were avoided (for example stoutness, body sythesis and bone mineral thickness). Fourteen examinations just talking about anticancer systems and eleven investigations without giving solid measures to disease were likewise prohibited. Three examinations considering the impact of specialists and three investigations with no suitable control were rejected.

At last, an aggregate of 59 creature contemplates satisfied the incorporation models. The attributes, significant results and methodological quality appraisal aftereffects of each investigation are given. Every one of the included examinations utilized malignancy murine models, aside from one investigation assessing epithelial ovarian disease (OVAC) preventive systems which utilized the chicken model. Unconstrained model, compound instigated model, transgenic model and relocated model were embraced by the included examinations. Two sorts of chemical touchy malignancies bosom disease and prostate disease were generally considered, trailed by cerebrum malignant growth and hepatic malignant growth. The scores of characteristics of the examinations utilizing STAIR went from 3 to 5.

Caloric Restriction and Cancer

Forty four included examinations that assessed antitumor impacts in creatures were set on CR. Among them, murine models were most oftentimes utilized (43 investigations) and chicken model was utilized in one examination. The most contemplated malignancy types were mammary, prostate, mind, pancreatic, and hepatic tumors. Skin, colonic, ovarian and intestinal malignant growths were additionally researched each in a couple of related investigations. Unconstrained model, compound initiated model, transgenic model and relocated model were applied. Forty of the 44 examinations (90.9%) upheld the positive anticancer part of CR regardless of the various estimations. Thirty examinations explored the part of CR on inception of malignancy, 26 of which tended to the preventive job of CR on disease commencement. Fourteen examinations investigated the impact of CR on movement and three of them were likewise on metastasis of disease, these examinations showed that CR regulated movement and metastasis of malignant growth. The most utilized estimation was tumor occurrence communicated in rate. Tumor development, tumor weight and different estimations were additionally applied. From the included investigations, CR would in general be related with diminished weight contrasting with the controls.

Intermittent caloric limitation (ICR) and persistent caloric limitation (CCR) were concentrated independently by seven investigations. The time of limitation went from multi week to three weeks in ICR, trailed by an equivalent season of taking care of at AL. Six of the seven investigations finished up obviously that ICR was more viable in tumor avoidance than CCR, while the leftover examination didn't indicate (information not appeared).

In addition, one investigation showed that late-beginning CR which means applying CR diet after a time of AL diet additionally hindered epithelial sore turn of events.

Ketogenic Diet and Cancer

Nine examinations investigated the connection between sugar limitation and disease. All investigations utilized the murine models. The contemplated tumors included prostate, mind, colonic, gastric and metastatic diseases. Relocated models were applied by every one of the elaborate investigations. Eight of the nine investigations (88.9%) upheld that carb limitation is defensive on malignancy. One investigation utilizing the subject model and colon disease showed that low carb diet couldn't hinder tumor development. Eight articles researched the job of KD on movement of malignancy, and seven of them held a positive end. One article investigated the job of KD on metastasis of malignancy and demonstrated the job is productive. Weight changes were not uniform among the elaborate investigations. The sythesis of starch in the examinations went from 0 to 20%. The significant outcomes were introduced as tumor development and tumor volume. A healthfully complete and financially accessible ketogenic diet was contemplated, and the two important examinations all got positive ends albeit one depended on confined sums.

14

Meta-analysis and Cancer

Tumor rate was the most regularly utilized result with explicit information (in 22 examinations). 21 of them were about CR. The crude information of each investigation with tumor occurrence were pooled in our examination. The arbitrary impact model was applied as heterogeneity existed. The pooled for CR was 0.20 comparative with the controls, and this showed that CR assumes a preventive part against malignancy.

1.3 Intermittent Fasting and Cancer

There are eight examinations about intermittent fasting IF and disease. The fasting time went from 24 to 72 hours. The murine models were utilized. The most considered tumor types were prostate and hepatic malignancies. Relocated model, synthetic prompted model and transgenic model were applied. Five of the eight examinations (62.5%) got positive end, two of them utilized fasting cycle (48 h) with no predefined intermittent time and late-beginning intermittent fasting. Three examinations researched the part of IF on inception of malignancy, and two of them showed the proficient job of intermittent fasting IF. Five examinations looked through the part of IF on movement of disease, and three of them upheld the positive end. Two examinations broke down both IF and CR, and IF was utilitarian in postponing tumor development albeit the impact was not clear as CR. Three examinations acquired an adverse end that intermittent fasting IF was not fundamentally defensive on disease. The weight changes were not uniform among the elaborate examinations.

In this investigation, we assessed the fifty nine creature exploratory examinations on dietary limitation regimens and dissected the information to consider parts of caloric limitation, ketogenic diet and intermittent fasting during inception, movement and metastasis of malignancy in creature models. Our examination shows that CR is preventive on malignant growths as about 91% of pertinent investigations support the end and the aftereffect of meta-examination is huge. Our discoveries additionally show that KD can forestall malignant growth in spite of the fact that there are no persuading pooled information. In any case, no enough proof shows the preventive impact of IF on malignancies.

A meta-examination on CR and unconstrained bosom tumors in subject somewhere in the range of 1942 and 1994 found that energy-limited creatures created 55% less bosom malignancies than the controls, which was like our discoveries zeroed in on investigations somewhere in the range of 1994 and 2014.

In spite of the fact that CR was emphatically connected with diminished malignant growth hazard in creature models, the impact in human is as yet unclear. It is practically difficult to survey the drawn out malignancy rate of solid individuals with CR diet. The current clinical preliminaries were most directed in corpulent disease patients, with biomarkers as the most distinguished file. Be that as it may, finishes of these clinical preliminaries were not generally the equivalent. In an examination exploring the impact of dietary mediation, the recently analyzed stout prostate disease patients were randomized to a CR diet bunch or a benchmark group and contrasts in weight reduction and insulin-like development factor (IGF) restricting proterin-3 (IGFBP-3) levels were found in the CR bunch. IGFBP-3 is the most plentiful IGFBP and serum level is emphatically connected with prostate malignancy. In an examination about large postmenopausal ladies, no critical changes of IGF-1 or IGFBP-3 were distinguished in the dietary-prompted weight reduction bunch, yet the proportion of IGF-1 or IGFBP-3 expanded in this mediation bunch, which were conflicting with another investigation or with the discoveries from creature tests. In a randomized controlled preliminary, the degrees of aggravation biomarkers were diminished in postmenopausal ladies with a CR weight reduction diet, and this outcome was significant as expanded degrees of incendiary biomarkers are related with expanded danger for certain malignant growths. Quality articulation in bosom tissue was likewise concentrated in corpulent ladies, just as stomach tissues, and huge changes were distinguished in glycolytic and lipid blend pathways following CR. What's more, quality included like (SCD) was discovered to be a vital factor in guideline of tumorigenesis in vivo.

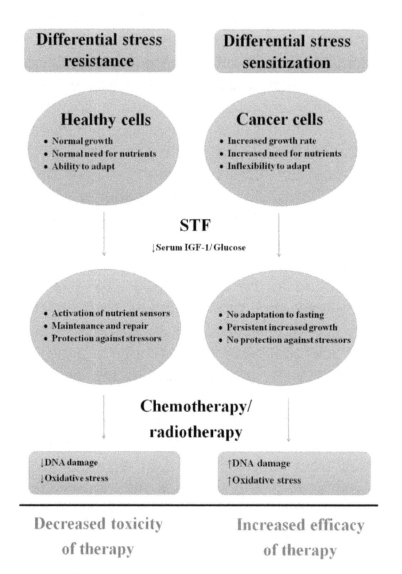

The included creature tests show that ICR is more successful than CCR in anticipation of diseases. A clinical preliminary contrasting ICR (2 days out of each week) and CCR in youthful overweight ladies showed that both

ICR and CCR included a 25% energy limitation. Then again, actually ICR was similarly successful for weight reduction as CCR, the progressions of numerous markers recognized like CPR, IGF-1, IGFBP-1, and IGPBP-2 were likewise comparable between the two gatherings. The investigation got an end that ICR might be an identical option in contrast to CCR for weight reduction and lessening infection hazard.

KD may likewise have extraordinary potential in malignancy anticipation in our investigation, which was upheld by eight of the nine included examinations. The connection among KD and malignant growth is indistinct in the clinical domain. One investigation looking at the impact of intermittent energy and starch limitation (40 g sugar for each d for 2 d each week) with day by day energy limitation in overweight ladies showed that the previous is better than the last in progress of insulin affectability and diminished muscle to fat ratio. Nonetheless, this examination was not straightforwardly identified with KD. Attempted to survey the impacts of ketogenic diet in two patients with cutting edge harmful astrocytoma tumors, the outcome that glucose take-up at the tumor site was decreased. A few existing clinical preliminaries distinguishing KD in the oncology populace are as yet continuous.

Intermittent fasting IF may not be an ideal dietary intercession in creature tests since 37.5% of the included examinations gave adverse outcomes. Nonetheless, the aftereffects of clinical analyses are hazy. A case arrangement report showed that fasting joined with chemotherapy is protected and may debilitate the chemotherapy-initiated results albeit just 10 cases were incorporated. In the exploration, patients willfully abstained for as long as 180 hours prior or potentially following chemotherapy. Fasting cycles joined with chemotherapy drugs were likewise concentrated in creature tests, and were powerful and could draw out disease free endurance. In any case, clinical information for intermittent fasting IF are meager, and some other existing clinical preliminaries surveying intermittent fasting IF in the oncology populace are as yet continued.

Notwithstanding, human experience for applying these dietary limitation regimens in disease counteraction is restricted. There are numerous deficiencies in the current clinical trials. Right off the bat, numerous investigations need control gatherings and reliabilities of these examinations are adequately not. Besides, the limitation regimens can't generally be endured by every one of the subjects through the examination. Thirdly, the exploration time frames are short, and the drawn out impacts of dietary regimens can't be very much clarified. Fourthly, the outcomes are frequently appeared as changes of biomarkers rather than direct proof.

1.4 Discussion

Besides, there are a few obstructions while in transit to utilize these dietary limitation regimens as a therapy or preventive mediation for disease. For instance, some dietary mediation strategies are unadherable over the long haul. Many results can be caused. Be that as it may, scientists are attempting to settle the difficulties to receive these dietary propensities into people. For instance, a powerful advanced way is CR mimetics, which can likewise assume an anticancer part like CR yet without requiring extraordinary energy limitation. IGF-1 pathways are expected significant arbiters in the anticancer capacity of CR, and pharmacologic mediations focused at these pathways are of extraordinary worth. An assortment of specialists will influence the pathways. A few specialists focusing at IGF-1 receptor like monoclonal antibodies and little atom tyrosine kinase inhibitors are under clinical preliminaries for some diseases.

Tentatively, the part of dietary limitation regimens against tumors in creature models has been concentrated broadly, yet the accomplishments have not been checked in people. Consequently, more clinical examinations are required. With respect to trouble in applying these dietary limitations into people, more passable regimens ought to be created. Since conditions contrast among malignancy patients, individualized treatment plan is important, so every tolerant can accomplish the best remedial impact. The frequency of ailing health is high in disease patients, and a few patients even experience the ill effects of cachexia. Therefore, dietary limitation treatment may be an issue for these patients as wholesome help is important. There ought to be a harmony between dietary limitation and healthful help. Endeavors ought to be made to completely examine the system of dietary regimens following up on tumors, and create specialists meddling with the pathways. Mimetics which can supplant dietary adjustments is an advancing expected territory.

In this examination, we inspected creature exploratory information of three dietary limitation regimens (CR, IF and KD) and pooled the open tumor occurrence information of CR. This examination has a few limits. In the first place, just analyses since 1994 were gathered, which may influence our decisions on the grounds that there are likewise some important examinations previously. Second, heterogeneity existed while pooling the information of CR, presumably because of the distinctions in creature models, malignancy types, test size, or perception time. Third, other information like tumor volume and endurance time were not pooled because of the modest number of pertinent examinations. Fourth, there are not many clinical tests, in this manner just creature tests were deliberately dissected.

Taking everything into account, the exploration shows that CR and KD are compelling in avoidance of malignancies in creature tests, yet the part of IF is farfetched. More clinical preliminaries are expected to research the viability and wellbeing of these dietary regimens. Dietary limitation routine which is more reasonable in human for disease counteraction and treatment ought to be distinguished. What's more, the important however more okay ways that can supplant dietary limitation ought to be additionally investigated.

Chapter 2. Impact of Intermittent Fasting on the Development of Prostate Cancer Tumor

Caloric limitation (CR) has been appeared to have hostile to malignant growth properties. Be that as it may, CR might be hard to apply in people auxiliary to consistence and possibly malicious impacts. An option is intermittent CR, or in the limit case intermittent fasting (IF). In a past little pilot study, we discovered 2 days out of each seven day stretch of IF with not obligatory benefiting from different days brought about patterns toward delayed endurance of subject bearing prostate malignancy xenografts. We tried to affirm these discoveries in a bigger report. A sum of 100 male serious joined immunodeficiency subject were infused subcutaneously with prostate disease cells. Subject were randomized to either not indispensable Western Diet (44% starches, 40% fat and 16% protein) or not obligatory Western Diet with twice-week by week twenty four hours diets (IF).

Tumor volumes and mouse bodyweights were estimated twice week after week. Subject were executed when tumor volumes came to 1000. Serum and tumor were gathered for examination of the insulin/insulin-like development factor 1 (IGF-1) hormonal pivot. In general, there was no distinction in mouse endurance or tumor volumes between gatherings. Mouse body loads were comparative between arms. Intermittent fasting IF subject had fundamentally higher serum IGF-1 levels and IGF-1 or IGFBP-3 proportions at executing. Be that as it may, no distinction was seen in serum insulin, IGFBP-3 or tumor levels. Intermittent fasting IF didn't improve mouse endurance nor did it defer prostate tumor development. This might be auxiliary to metabolic variations to the whole day fasting time frames. Future examinations are needed to advance CR for application in people.

2.1 Introduction

Caloric limitation (CR), under sustenance without hunger, is the solitary exploratory methodology reliably appeared to delay endurance in creature models. What's more, CR defers the advancement old enough related, obsessive sequalae and may drag out life, yet upgrade personal satisfaction. In little restricted common investigations in people and epidemiological examinations, momentary CR may decrease the rate old enough related infections including cardiovascular sickness and malignancy. Albeit these perceptions give a reasoning to preliminaries utilizing CR to forestall infections among more established individuals, exemplary CR is hard to carry out for an enormous scope because of helpless adherence. Besides, outrageous long haul CR may prompt other unexpected problems including over the top loss of muscle and fat mass. Accordingly, elective systems are expected to copy the medical advantages of exemplary CR regimens yet that are mediocre and effortlessly embraced by more established individuals.

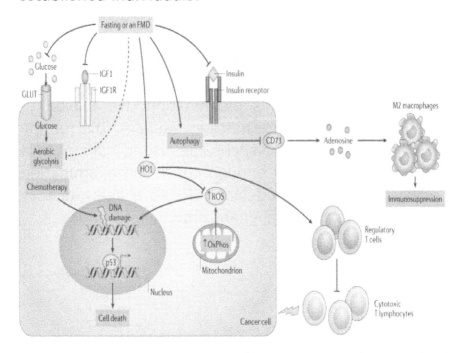

An option in contrast to what in particular might be portrayed as persistent CR is intermittent caloric limitation (ICR). We recently estimated that ICR may have a few, if not the entirety of the medical advantages of exemplary CR. To test this, we recently led a pilot concentrate in which 15 subject for each gathering were subcutaneously infused with LAPC-4 prostate malignancy tumor cells and took care of either not obligatory, as indicated by two exemplary CR regimens or one of four ICR regimens. In particular, the ICR routine that we tried was a proof-of-rule outrageous type of ICR: intermittent fasting (IF). Albeit a few of the IF and exemplary CR regimens were related with patterns toward delayed endurance, none arrived at importance in that restricted pilot study. Be that as it may, the most encouraging routine was taking care of subject not obligatory 5 days out of each week with two separate twenty four hours times of fasting each week. Strangely, subject in that gathering had patterns toward postponed tumor development without any distinctions in body weight, proposing that the advantages of IF may vary from those of exemplary CR. In this examination, we looked to explicitly test this intermittent fasting IF routine comparative with not indispensable taking care of in a bigger and all the more enough controlled examination to research IF, as a model of ICR, as a likely dietary mediation in prostate malignant growth.

Tumor Sample Study

Subsequent to acquiring endorsement from the Institutional Care and Use Committees, we got 100 male extreme joined immunodeficiency 7-to 8-week-old subject and housed 5 subject for each pen. At multi week before infusion, all subject were taken care of not obligatory Western Diet (40% fat, 44% sugars and 16% protein) arranged by Test Diet. Subject were infused subcutaneously in the correct flank with LAPC-4 tumor cells. At the point when tumors got discernible, tumor measurements were estimated with the utilization of calipers. Tumor volumes were determined utilizing the recipe. Both body loads and tumor volumes were estimated twice week after week. At the point when tumor volumes came to 200, subject were randomized to one of two investigation arms: not indispensable Western Diet (no mediation) or not obligatory Western Diet with twice week after week twenty four hours fasting periods (IF; abstained Monday and Thursday). After each fasting period, urinary ketones of subject in both investigation arms were acquired utilizing delicate supra pubic pressing factor and estimated utilizing semi quantitative pee ketone strips. At the point when tumors volumes arrived at 1000 or mouse wellbeing had all the earmarks of being undermined, subject were abstained for three hours then anesthetized and went through necropsy. At the hour of killing, the liver, prostate and xenograft tumor were gathered. Liver and prostate were snap frozen for future examinations. Tumors were separated with half being snap frozen and the rest of in 10% nonpartisan cradle formalin short-term and afterward implanted in paraffin. Mouse serum was gotten via cardiovascular cut and put away until investigated. Serum from the middle enduring 12 subject in each gathering was investigated for murine insulin, insulin-like development factor 1 (IGF-1) and IGFBP-3 levels utilizing chemical connected immunoassays.

Analysis of AKT

Tumor tests from the middle enduring 12 subject for each gathering were dissected for intracellular substance of (p-AKT), all out AKT (t-AKT) and beta-actin. LAPC-4 tumor lysates were readied utilizing the Mammalian Protein Preparation unit. Tests were homogenized in ice and centrifuged at forteen thousand grams for half hour. Protein focus in the supernatant part was resolved and separates were put away at short degrees. Protein groups were settled by sodium dodecyl sulfate polyacrylamide gel electrophoresis and immunoblots were created with ECL Plus reagent. Antibodies to p-AKT, t-AKT and beta-actin were gotten from Cell Signaling Technology. Protein groups were measured by densitometry examination utilizing Images (NIH).

Analysis of Stats

Examinations of tumor volumes, body loads and serum chemical levels between bunches were performed utilizing rank-aggregate test. Mouse endurance was looked at between arms utilizing the log-rank test and relative perils model. Endurance was graphically outlined utilizing bends. All measurable examinations were performed with a 0.05 cutoff for factual importance.

2.3 Results

Body Weight

As the two gatherings were not obligatory taken care of when not fasting, no endeavor to quantify caloric admission was made. Notwithstanding, regardless of the IF bunch just approaching food 5 days of the week, we noticed no critical contrasts in subject body loads between the two arms whenever point.

Tumor Growth

Generally, there were no critical contrasts between bunches in tumor volume whenever point. At the hour of randomization (day 0), tumor volumes in the not obligatory took care of gathering were like those in the intermittent fasting IF bunch. At the later time focuses, there was an idea of bigger tumors in the IF bunch, however this didn't arrive at measurable importance. At the hour of killing, last tumor volumes were discovered to be comparative between study arms. Also, in general endurance characterized as time from randomization to killing was not diverse between arms.

Urinary Ketones and Serum Glucose

In the event that subject had altogether higher urinary ketone levels contrasted and the not obligatory gathering after the main fasting time frames. Notwithstanding, despite the fact that ketone levels stayed higher in the IF bunch for the initial six fasting cycles, they bit by bit declined in the IF gathering with the end goal that by the seventh and past fasting scenes, there were no critical contrasts between the gatherings in urinary ketone levels. Urinary ketone levels at the hour of killing were comparable between gatherings. At the hour of killing, not obligatory subject had a fundamentally higher fasting serum glucose levels in contrast with intermittent fasting IF subject.

Hormone Levels

Serum insulin and IGFBP-3 levels were comparable between study gatherings. Interestingly, intermittent fasting IF subject had a roughly 48% higher middle degree of IGF-1 than not indispensable subject. Additionally, middle IGF-1 or IGFBP-3 proportion levels were likewise altogether higher in the IF arm comparative with those in the not obligatory gathering.

Total and Activated ATK

Phosphorylated, or initiated, AKT is a downstream atomic marker of IGF-1 chemical action as well as being a free indicator of prostate malignant growth movement and repeat. Accordingly, we tried to measure the overall degrees of AKT initiation in tumor cell lysate by western blotch. There was no contrasts between the gatherings in the degrees of actuated or t-AKT or in the proportion of enacted t-AKT.

2.4 Discussion

Diet is likely a significant factor in both disease advancement and movement. In particular, expanded caloric admission animates tumor development while CR lessens both the rate of malignancy and its movement across different creature models. Anyway optional to helpless consistence and injurious results from outrageous CR (that is, loss of bulk and weight), human preliminaries may not mirror the promising outcomes saw in creature contemplates. To conquer these likely impediments, we and others have proposed ICR as a way to get the medical advantages of CR that would possibly be more adequate to patients. Already in a pilot study, we discovered an idea that IF (twice week by week twenty four hours fasting periods with not obligatory benefiting from re-took care of days) as a proof of standard in regards to ICR may postpone prostate tumor development without decreases in body weight. Thus, we tried to approve this IF methodology as a dietary mediation to defer tumor development and movement in a bigger, all around fueled investigation. We tracked down that comparative with not indispensable taking care of, IF through twice-week after week twenty four hours fasting periods with not obligatory benefiting from re-took care of days didn't defer tumor development nor did it present an endurance benefit to subject embedded with LAPC-4 xenografts. Likewise, intermittent fasting IF was incapable in down directing the insulin/IGF-1 pivot, a critical instrument through which CR eases back tumor development. These discoveries propose that twice week after week IF doesn't regulate tumor science adequately to repress tumor development.

CR has been appeared to improve the length and personal satisfaction of vertebrate and invertebrate creatures the same. All the more as of late, CR has shown anticancer properties in different malignant growth models. It is imagined that CR shows this anticancer impact through a large number of pathways including decrease of muscle versus fat as well as weight, diminished age of free extremists and balance of key cell pathways. In particular, one pathway well modified by CR is the insulin or IGF-1 hormonal hub. This hub has been both epidemiologically and tentatively connected to the turn of events and movement of prostate malignant growth. Regardless of the guarantee of CR, there are sure hindrances that conceivably meddle with its relevance in people. As most constant CR regimens require decrease of caloric admission for broadened timeframes, consistence stays an issue. Loss of muscle to fat ratio as well as weight is generally seen as one of the advantages to CR. Be that as it may, for men with late stage infection in whom counteraction of cachexia is a key objective, weight reduction may not be alluring.

To make CR more tasteful, examiners have endeavored to catch every one of the advantages of decreased caloric admission while limiting its adverse consequences. One proposed method of achieving this might be ICR. It is discovered that exposing subject to 2-week exchanging times of half CR followed by permitting the subject to eat 100% of the calories devoured by age-coordinated with control subject brought about postponed prostate tumor discovery and improved endurance comparative with both not indispensable taking care of and nonstop CR. In a later cross-sectional examination by a similar gathering, there was an idea that a similar 2-week substituting ICR approach was better than 25% persistent CR in its capacity to defer prostate tumor location. In our own past experience we adopted an alternate strategy and instead of utilizing fourteen days of half CR followed by re-feeding at 100%, we zeroed in on short exceptional times of outrageous CR (that is, fasting) and afterward took into account either not obligatory or isocaloric admission on re-fed days. Patterns were seen for an estimated 40% improvement in endurance in subject that were abstained twice week by week and permitted unhindered admittance to benefit from re-fed days. Furthermore, this idea that twice week by week fasting diminished mortality was done without weight reduction. Notwithstanding, this past investigation was a pilot study and the outcomes were not genuinely huge with just subject per arm, and accordingly, these discoveries required approval in a bigger report before human preliminaries.

Generally speaking, we discovered no distinction in mouse endurance. This differences with the discoveries of specialist wherein ICR, yet conveyed utilizing an alternate convention, did essentially drag out endurance. It is important that, reliable with our pilot information and rather than the information, there was no weight reduction among the IF subject in this investigation. This is because of the way that on no fasting days, subject were taken care of not indispensable, permitting them to gorge, checking the fasting, and bringing about no net body weight change. This is a central issue of qualification between our investigation and that of specialist wherein in the last examination ICR was conveyed in 2-week times of half CR followed by re-taking care of, yet restricting admission to 100% old enough coordinated with subject in the not indispensable arm, subsequently forestalling overloading. Taken together, these information imply that ICR without weight reduction has no advantage. On the other hand, within the sight of weight reduction, ICR seems to have benefits far in excess of those of persistent CR. Eventually, regardless of whether the contrasts between the current and past ICR examines are identified with the presence or nonattendance of weight reduction, and additionally the term/seriousness of CR in the ICR regimens (that is, twenty four hours quick versus 2-week half CR) or some other factor stays to be resolved.

It is additionally tracked down that intermittent fasting IF successfully brought down articulation of the insulin/IGF-1 hormonal pivot. Anyway in this examination, both IGF-1 levels and IGF-1/IGFBP-3 proportions were fundamentally expanded in ICR subject contrasted and not indispensable subject, while serum insulin and IGFBP-3 levels were comparative. It very well might be conceivable that raised IGF-1 levels in IF subject are the outcome of overloading on re-took care of days. In a new critique, features a few investigations that partner unreasonable caloric admission with rises in IGF-1. In any case, scientist alerts that as of now the information don't totally show how much key hormonal tomahawks are adjusted by overloading auxiliary to potential between and intra-species contrasts in endocrine reaction to abundance calories. At the point when we inspected p-AKT, t-AKT and p-AKT/t-AKT proportions, a marker of downstream IGF-1 action, no distinction was found between gatherings. We propose this absence of expanded downstream movement notwithstanding raised IGF-1 levels can be clarified by the impact of fasting on other IGFBPs beside IGFBP-3. In particular, IGFBP-1 and IGFBP-2 have been proposed to be inhibitors of IGF-1 and are discovered to be expanded during seasons of delayed diets. Accordingly we conjecture that notwithstanding rises IGF-1 in IF, expected expansions in inhibitory IGFBPs may have quieted the effect of the raised serum IGF-1 on tumor science. Then again, the slight contrasts in IGF-1 might not have been huge enough to defeat different factors, for example, the comparable body loads and insulin levels.

We analyzed urinary ketones to gauge energy substrate use without dietary glucose (that is, when abstained). We found that however intermittent fasting IF subject at first had fundamentally higher ketone levels than not obligatory subject, with each progressive quick, IF subject turned out to be dynamically less ketotic eventually moving toward urinary ketone levels saw in not indispensable subject. IGF-1 has been proposed to decidedly affect serum glucose control. We theorize that expanded degrees of IGF-1 in IF subject served to work with improved glucose take-up. This slow improvement in glucose take-up could be reflected by diminished urinary ketone levels, as found in this examination. This 'standardization' of urinary ketone levels could reflect improved glucose use by the host and potentially the tumor. Thusly, it stays conceivable the negative discoveries from this examination come from the mouse's capacity to adjust to twenty four hours fasting periods by directing its digestion, however this requires further investigation. Regardless of whether longer fasting periods with ostensible food admission would have benefits without weight reduction stays to be resolved.

One limit to our investigation is the utilization of a murine prostate malignant growth model. As these creatures have generally better abilities to burn calories contrasted with people, we figured the effect of the twenty four hours diets would be more articulated. In any case, our information recommend that the subject digestion systems were above and beyond to conquer brief fasting periods. Also, how much this verification of-guideline way to deal with outrageous ICR (that is, IF) would be feasible in people is obscure. Nonetheless, the negative information from this investigation don't uphold further testing and at last further examinations are expected to all the more likely refine CR and ICR conventions to moderate prostate disease development.

Chapter 3. Intermittent Fasting Reduce Cancer Rates in Overweight Patients

Creature studies and human observational information connect energy limitation (ER) to decreased paces of carcinogenesis. The majority of these examinations have included consistent energy limitation (CER), however there is expanding public and logical interest in the possible wellbeing and anticancer impacts of intermittent energy limitation (IER) or intermittent fasting (IF), which involve times of stamped ER or complete fasting blended with times of ordinary eating. This audit sums up creature considers that surveyed tumor rates with IER and IF contrasted and CER or not indispensable feed utilization. The significance of these creature information to human malignant growth is additionally considered by summing up accessible human investigations of the impacts of IER or IF contrasted and CER on disease biomarkers in large, overweight, and ordinary weight subjects. IER regimens that incorporate times of ER substituting with not indispensable feed utilization for 1, 2, or multi week have been accounted for to be better than CER in diminishing tumor rates in many unconstrained subject tumor models. Restricted human information from momentary investigations in overweight and fat subjects have shown that IER can prompt more prominent enhancements in insulin affectability (homeostasis model appraisal) than can CER, with practically identical decreases in adipokines and fiery markers and minor changes in the insulin-like development factor hub. There are at present no information contrasting IER or IF and CER in ordinary weight subjects. The advantages of IER in these momentary preliminaries are of interest, however not adequate proof to suggest the utilization of IER above CER. Longer-term human investigations of adherence to and adequacy and wellbeing of IER are needed in stout and overweight subjects, just as should be expected weight subjects.

3.1 Introduction

Overabundance adiposity and over sustenance are significant reasons for malignant growth. An increment in BMI of 5 is related with a 20–52% more serious danger of 13 tumors, including endometrial, nerve bladder, renal, rectal, postmenopausal bosom, pancreatic, thyroid, colon, and esophageal diseases; leukemia; various myeloma; non-Hodgkin lymphoma; and dangerous melanoma. Biomarker-aligned energy admission is decidedly connected with absolute malignant growth, just as with bosom, colon, endometrial, and kidney disease in postmenopausal ladies. Observational proof shows that weight decrease with energy limitation (ER) lessens the danger of bosom malignancy, while weight decrease with bariatric medical procedure diminishes the danger of disease, basically in ladies.

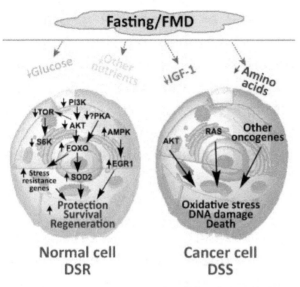

Trends in Endocrinology & Metabolism

Diminished tumor advancement with ER was first distinguished in an investigation by Rous, which exhibited that ER deferred the improvement of repeat and the development of mammary tumors in subject. 100 years of resulting lab research has affirmed that ER forestalls tumor improvement in rodents, and numerous examinations demonstrate that ER draws out the life expectancy. The comparator bunches in these examinations were mostly overloaded, stationary research center creatures. In this manner, these examinations demonstrate that ER can lessen the disease advancing impacts of stoutness and over sustenance, however these discoveries may not have any significant bearing to ordinary weight creatures or human subjects, for whom ER might be inadequate or potentially unfavorable.

The significance of the kind of control in randomized investigations of ER was exhibited in 2 continuous long haul primate considers. The Wisconsin National Primate Research Center investigation showed that a 20–25% day by day or nonstop energy limitation (CER) decreased diabetes and cardiovascular infection (CVD) contrasted and control creatures burning-through feed not obligatory. Notwithstanding, these illnesses were not decreased in 20–25% CER-took care of monkeys in a National Institute on Aging (NIA) study contrasted and moderately lighter controls that got controlled as opposed to not indispensable segments of food. Hence, the information in the Wisconsin study recommended that ER decreased the danger of diabetes and CVD when it conquered the unfavorable impacts of over sustenance and abundance adiposity, yet the information in the NIA study proposed that ER didn't have these impacts in lighter rhesus monkeys. Curiously, the 20–25% CER prompted equivalent decreases in disease rates in the two examinations. Malignant growth rates for ER and control in the Wisconsin National Primate Research Center investigation were 4 and 8, separately; in the NIA study, rates were 0 and 6, individually. In this way, a 25% CER had anticancer impacts in lighter just as heavier rhesus monkeys.

Most ER research has included CER. Choices incorporate intermittent energy limitation (IER) or intermittent fasting (IF), which includes times of stamped ER or absolute fasting mixed with times of typical eating. These methodologies as of late have gotten a lot of logical and public interest. This inexorably mainstream dietary methodology is simply the subject of many assistance books that guarantee that this example of eating is ideal for weight reduction, decreasing infirmity, and advancing life span. The fascination of IER above standard CER approaches is the statement that IER can apply advantageous wellbeing impacts when weight and complete energy admission are kept up. These helpful impacts are asserted for ordinary load just as overweight people. Be that as it may, these cases for human medical advantages are extrapolations of information from creature concentrates in which IER regimens regularly delivered a general ER, and diminished weight and adiposity contrasted and overweight controls who devoured food not obligatory.

The increased logical and public interest in IER and its reception by various overweight and typical weight subjects overall methods existing information should be summed up. Early IER analysts, cautioned of the risks "that exploration discoveries might be combined with ideas and estimates to develop ideas which by pyramided reiteration become acknowledged."

This survey article will sum up creature investigations of tumor improvement with IER or IF contrasted and CER and their relative impacts on key markers of tumorigenesis. The pertinence of these creature information to human disease is considered by summing up accessible human investigations of the impacts of IER or IF contrasted and CER on malignant growth hazard biomarkers in fat, overweight, and ordinary weight subjects.

Specialist first announced that intermittent fasting IF in quite a while (no food on substitute days, scattered with long stretches of ordinary eating) expanded life span by 15–20% and diminished mammary tumor development by 65–90% contrasted and those burning-through feed not indispensable. Decreases were corresponding to the quantity of long stretches of fasting each week and the measure of weight decrease. A few exploratory intermittent taking care of conventions in creatures have been concentrated from that point forward that included times of IF (most generally substitute long stretches of all out food hardship) or IER. The most-contemplated regimens in people have been substitute day fasting (ADF) or IER, with either 2 continuous days out of each week, or substitute day energy limitation (ADER), commonly 75%. The expression "intermittent fasting" is utilized in the writing to depict times of either no admission (i.e., IF) or diminished admission (i.e., IER). Nonetheless, there are likely unique metabolic and organic reactions among IF and IER. For instance, there might be more noteworthy metabolic variances during fasting periods and hyperphagia during non-confined periods with IF than with IER. We characterized intermittent fasting IF as times of no admission and a total ER, and IER as intermittent times of diminished food consumption and a halfway ER. We will sum up information for IF and IER independently.

The audit will address the accompanying 4 key inquiries and feature regions for additional examination: 1) Do IER and IF achieve decreases in tumor rates when they accomplish a general ER or without a general ER, and how does this contrast and CER? 2) Do IER and IF effect malignant growth hazard biomarkers in people when they accomplish a general ER or without a general ER, and how does this contrast and CER? 3) Do IER and IF have malignant growth defensive impacts in ordinary load just as fat/overweight subjects? 4) Are IER and IF safe, or could they have possible unfriendly impacts in hefty/overweight and ordinary weight subjects?

3.3 Effect of Intermittent Fasting on Tumors

Tumor models

An assortment of IF regimens have been tried, going from substitute long stretches of fasting to infrequent times of five days of fasting. On the off chance that regimens decreased mammary tumor rates by 40–80% contrasted and not indispensable utilization. The antitumor impact of IF in these investigations is relative to the level of generally ER and decreased body weight contrasted and the gathering burning-through not indispensable. Whenever didn't effect mammary or prostate tumors when subject were permitted to overload on unlimited days and their general energy admission coordinated with the energy admission of the gathering burning-through feed not obligatory. The IF subject in one of these prostate tumor contemplates had higher serum insulin-like development factor (IGF) I focuses than did the subject devouring feed not indispensable, however they didn't have expanded downstream protein kinase B flagging.

revealed that insufficient subject undertaking 1 day of food hardship each week (25% weight decrease) had diminished paces of neoplasms (essentially sarcoma) and a transitional endurance that was not exactly those on a day by day ER and more noteworthy than the gathering that burned-through feed not obligatory. It is accounted for that 2 days of intermittent fasting each week and not indispensable eating for 5 days with no general ER decreased the movement of lung, ovarian, and hepatic human xenografts in a safe traded off mouse model. These decreases were related with diminished IGF-I, megakaryocyte development and platelet creation, and expanded characteristic executioner action. The significance of this finding to human malignancies isn't known.

IER has been concentrated chiefly in mouse models at the college. Mammary tumor examines tried patterns of 3 weeks of half ER (for the most part starch limitation) and 3 weeks not obligatory utilization. Four examinations in estrogen-responsive mouse mammary tumor infection subject all discovered IER to be better than not obligatory utilization. IER was better than isoenergetic CER in 3 of these examinations, and equivalent in study. Two extra examinations were led in a human epidermal development factor receptor 2 estrogen–inert tumor model. One investigation discovered IER to be identical to CER, and the two eating regimens decreased tumor rates contrasted and a not indispensable eating routine. Be that as it may, the subsequent investigation, which utilized a similar model, didn't discover huge contrasts in tumor rates between IER, CER, and not indispensable utilization.

In this manner, an IER with 3 weeks of substitute ER and not indispensable utilization might be same or better than a comparable CER for conquering the tumor-advancing impacts of over nourishment in subject inclined to creating estrogen receptor–positive MMTV-actuated mammary tumors. The more noteworthy impacts of IER contrasted and CER recommends that IER is applying extra malignancy defensive impacts notwithstanding the impacts of diminished weight. Conversely, the estrogen receptor negative tumor model shows up less receptive to ER, with same and unassuming impacts of IER and CER. Ovarian cycling chemicals were not evaluated in these examinations. Different researchers found that both 25% CER and 7 days of half ER could prevent feminine cycling in subject, resulting in significant decreases in estrogen, which could explain the benefits of IER and CER in estrogen-responsive mouse models.

The scientist bunch likewise considered the impacts of IER on the improvement of prostate malignant growth in a transgenic adenocarcinoma mouse prostate model. An IER routine that elaborate fourteen days of half ER (basically starch limitation) and fourteen days of controlled not indispensable utilization (a by and large 25% ER) didn't impact prostate malignancy rates. In any case, IER expanded opportunity to-tumor discovery and endurance contrasted and not obligatory utilization and an isoenergetic CER, alongside related more noteworthy decreases in serum IGF-I and leptin and higher serum adiponectin. A comparative investigation of IER (multi week of half ER and multi week of controlled not obligatory utilization) in pancreatic malignant growth inclined subject announced less pancreatic injuries with IER than with isoenergetic CER and not indispensable feed utilization. The component of this impact isn't known, yet it has all the earmarks of being free of IGF-I and the mammalian objective of pathway action, which diminished in the CER however not in the IER bunch.

Tumor caused by Carcinogen

CER decreased tumor rates in various cancer-causing agent actuated tumor models. Conversely, IER and intermittent fasting IF had all the earmarks of being impeding, and could build tumor rates on the off chance that they were started inside about a month of cancer-causing agent openness, i.e., during the basic disease advancement stage. IER didn't have the malignancy defensive impacts of CER with cancer-causing agent incited mammary, hepatic, and colorectal tumors in rodents. Revealed a 12% expanded pace of mammary tumors in rodents with IER contrasted and not indispensable feed utilization, in spite of a by and large 14% ER contrasted and the gathering that devoured feed not obligatory. In like manner, intermittent fasting IF expanded tumor rates in rodents contrasted and not indispensable feed utilization in cancer-causing agent prompted models of colon and liver tumors. Interestingly, presentation of IER and IF 4 two months after cancer-causing agent openness in rodents decreased mammary carcinomas by half and the advancement of liver sores by 65% contrasted and not obligatory feed utilization.

Summary of intermittent Fasting on Subject Models

In the event that has been contrasted and not obligatory taking care of in subjects. Whenever diminished tumor rates and tumor development essentially when there was a general ER and decreased bodyweight. Whenever didn't conquer the malignancy advancing impacts of over sustenance in most of creature models when weight and generally energy admission were kept up.

IER regimens that included exchanging times of ER and not indispensable feed utilization for 1, 2 or 3 weeks have been accounted for to be better than CER in defeating the tumor-advancing impacts of over nourishment in some yet not all creature tumor models. The more prominent disease defensive impacts of IER contrasted and CER recommend that IER applied extra consequences for these diminished weight creatures; consequently, there are likely advantages for IER in ordinary weight creatures and subjects. IER and IF started at the hour of cancer-causing agent organization was not viable, though it was successful whenever given a month after organization of the cancer-causing agent. The importance of cancer-causing agent initiated tumors to the human circumstance isn't clear, however it shows that IER and IF regimens may not offer disease insurance in all circumstances.

Proliferation of Cell

Decreased expansion in epithelial cells could diminish malignant growth commencement and the resulting advancement of started tumor cells. A constant ER of 25–30% has evoked stamped decreases in mammary epithelial cell expansion in subject, which isn't seen with more modest day by day limitations, e.g., a 5% CER. Mammary and prostate cell multiplication has been diminished with ADF or an adequately limited ADER routine (85% limitation on confined days). Mammary cell expansion was decreased with both a 85% ADER and an ADF contrasted and not indispensable utilization, however not with a 75% ADER. Strangely, decreases in expansion with these regimens were similar with decreases accomplished with a 25% CER, yet they were accomplished without forcing a general ER and without lessening body weight. Essentially, decreases in prostate cell multiplication were accounted for with a 85% ADER or ADF, yet were not seen with a half ADER.

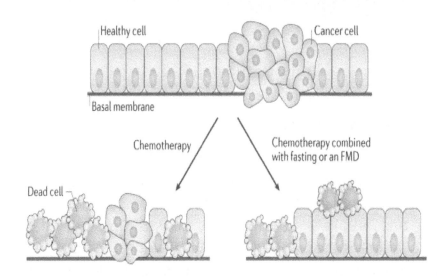

The decreased cell expansion rates in these examinations were accounted for on the morning following the hyperphagic not obligatory day of ADER or ADF. This recommends that IER has a supported impact on multiplication during both confined and not indispensable days, given that there is an adequately extreme limitation on limited days. Notwithstanding, IER and IF creatures devour their day by day energy consumption inside a couple of hours on devouring days, making a more prominent self-inflicted time of no food admission before the estimations, which may represent a portion of the decreases in expansion noticed.

CER diminishes mammary cell multiplication in rodents, to a great extent by loss of estrous cycle, decreases in regenerative chemical fixations, and diminished IGF-I focuses. Estrous cycles were unaffected in subject going through ADER or ADF. Diminished mammary and prostate cell expansion in these examinations has happened close by decreased serum IGF-I focuses. The significance of these information to the human circumstance isn't known, on the grounds that the impacts of IER and IF on human IGF-I action are not all around described. Presently, as far as anyone is concerned, there are no human information on the impacts of IER, IF, and CER on cell expansion.

Resistance against Stress

Emergency room is thought to lessen the danger of malignant growths and different sicknesses to some degree through hormesis, whereby ER goes about as a low-force stressor that evokes cytoprotective impacts by means of versatile up guideline of cell stress obstruction pathways. These pathways incorporate up guideline of kinases and deacetylases, including sirtuins, protein chaperones that arrange protein combination, collapsing, disaggregation, and debasement; cancer prevention agents; chemicals; and autophagy. In rodents, ADF has been demonstrated to be a compelling type of ER in lessening tissue harm in the mind and heart contrasted and not obligatory utilization, and has been discovered to be better than CER in securing hippocampal neurons against energize poisonous injury.

Autophagy is accounted for to be fleetingly up controlled during the initial 24 hours of fasting in rat liver, muscle, kidney, and heart, part of the way in light of expanded ketones. The impacts of fasting on autophagy inside the more extensive scope of target tissues in people influenced by malignant growth have not been contemplated. Besides, the job of autophagy in the advancement of human diseases in various tissues is mind boggling and not obvious.

Antioxidant Activity and Oxidative Stress

Oxidative pressure is connected to the advancement of malignancy and sped up maturing, with the overall theory being that receptive oxygen species creation ought to be restricted to diminish cell harm. A new change in outlook has featured the way that ROS creation might be needed to inspire a compulsory gentle cell stress reaction, which thusly up manages cancer prevention agent pathways and brings down by and large long haul oxidative pressure. In this manner, changes in cancer prevention agent protein movement with IER or IF, particularly when creatures have adjusted to expand their chemical action, may give a more pertinent marker of their effect on illness hazard than ROS creation in essence.

In male rodents, a month of ADF with rotating 24 hours of absolute food hardship and 24 hours of hyperphagia (150% not indispensable admission) and 14% by and large ER didn't influence cancer prevention agent chemical action (glutathione peroxidase, glutathione reductase, or catalase) in the heart or liver after hyperphagic feed days, however prompted diminished movement of catalase in the cerebrum and glutathione peroxidase in muscle contrasted and rodents that devoured a not obligatory eating routine. These rodents experienced expanded convergences of certain (carbonyls) yet not all (protein nitration) oxidative harm markers in the cerebrum and liver. A prior investigation from this gathering, notwithstanding, announced huge expansions in cancer prevention agent compound action in muscle and fat tissue following a more drawn out term

32 weeks openness to IF (estimated after feed days) contrasted and isoenergetic not obligatory feed utilization. Announced that four months of ADF in subject expanded superoxide dismutase action in the mind, spleen, and mitochondria, yet decreased superoxide dismutase action in the liver contrasted and isoenergetic not obligatory feed utilization. In this manner, intermittent fasting IF seemed to effect cell reinforcement limit in various tissues. Chemical action may increment with longer openness to IF as a drawn out variation in light of the underlying expansion in oxidative pressure with IF.

The impact of changes in cell reinforcement protein exercises on the real improvement of malignant growth is hazy. Expanded cell reinforcement catalyst movement, alongside decreased ROS creation, in intermittent fasting IF subject contrasted and those devouring not obligatory feed meant diminished lymphoma rate. (0% for intermittent fasting IF contrasted and 33% for controls that devoured not obligatory feed). In any case, it is accounted for that multi week of a 20% CER in rodents decreased mammary organ oxidative DNA harm by 25% contrasted and not indispensable utilization, though an IER that was isoenergetic to the CER bunch (5 patterns of about a month and a half of half IER and fourteen days of get up to speed hyperphagia at 150% not obligatory admission) expanded DNA harm by 30%. In this way, there is a potential for unfriendly impacts with IER. Weight reduction preliminaries of IER contrasted and CER in overweight/large premenopausal ladies have shown conflicting consequences for cutting edge oxidative protein items. One examination revealed equivalent 20%

decreases with both IER and CER. A subsequent report revealed no adjustment of cutting edge oxidative protein items with one or the other methodology.

Problems investigating Intermittent Fasting in Subjects and their relevance to Human Cancers

The most convincing information to help explicit decreases in tumors with IER are rat considers, which have announced diminished tumor rates contrasted and rates in consistently took care of creatures, regardless of obviously equivalent body loads and energy consumption. Nonetheless, similar weight, IER, IF, and consistently took care of creatures could have various sums and conveyance of muscle versus fat, which are not frequently estimated. Numerous creature contemplates are probably going to be underpowered to survey unassuming contrasts in energy consumption that may exist among IER and CER gatherings.

The unfavorable impacts of IER and IF in some creature models might be the aftereffect of hyperphagia on non-confined days. Then again, times of fasting with IF or energy or sugar limitation with IER summon floods in lipolysis and fat oxidation and expansions in coursing FFAs and ketone bodies, which could be inconvenient. Expanded FFAs and ketones have been connected to the development of specific tumors. Fasting for 1–7 days expanded coursing FFAs 5-to 7-overlap and ketone bodies 20-overlay, which was related with the development of Walker carcinoma 256 and Jensen sarcoma in rodents.

These expected unfriendly impacts of fasting and ER in creature models are imperative to consider, yet may not be an issue for people. Interestingly with creature considers, compensatory overloading isn't found in human investigations. IER (2 continuous d/week) prompted a 20–30% ER and not hyperphagia on unhindered days in investigations of overweight and hefty people. Moreover, ADER was related with a 5% ER on unlimited days in fat subjects.

The high motions in flowing FFAs and ketone bodies connected to diminished development chemical creation seen with fasting and ER in rodents are not found in people, especially not in hefty subjects who have decreased development chemical creation contrasted and slender subjects. A 36 hours complete quickly in corpulent and slender subjects expanded coursing FFAs by 1.7-and 2.4-overlap, separately, and ketone bodies by 6-and 18-overlay, individually. Fasting actuates more quick ascents in FFAs and ketones in ladies than in men. IER is probably going to summon a lot more modest motion in FFAs and ketones than is intermittent fasting IF. In our own examinations, IER (2 days of 75% ER) prompted a little (20%) increment in serum ketones and a 10–300% expansion in groupings of individual FFAs on the morning after the 2 limited day.

Study of Intermittent Fasting in Obese

There are no information, as far as anyone is concerned, on the impacts of IER and IF on malignant growth rates in people. Here, we sum up accessible human information contrasting the impacts of IER and IF with CER on disease hazard biomarkers that are thought to intercede the connections among adiposity and energy consumption and the turn of events and development of malignant growths, including insulin, IGF-I, leptin, adiponectin, cytokines, and irritation related atoms. Since numerous biomarkers are probably going to have stamped intense changes during limited and taking care of days of the IER, we have possibly announced this information when the day of estimation (taking care of or fasting) has been determined, consequently giving a precise portrayal of the generally metabolic impacts of the IER and intermittent fasting IF regimens. Discoveries are accounted for independently for large and overweight subjects and for ordinary weight subjects.

3.5 Effect of Intermittent Fasting on Metabolic Cancer Risk Markers

Insulin sensitivity, GF-I and Insulin

Checked decreases in serum IGF-I are thought to intercede the disease defensive impacts of CER, IER, and intermittent fasting IF in rat considers. Interestingly, coursing groupings of all out IGF-I and bioactive IGF-I [determined by insulin-like development factor restricting protein (IGFBP) 1, IGFBP-2, and IGFBP-3] have all the earmarks of being helpless markers of the impacts of ER and weight reduction in people. Serum IGF-I frequently increments close by weight reduction, ER, and work out, and is contrarily connected to general adiposity and hepatic fat. Serum IGF-I fixations don't relate well to IGF-I bioactivity inside tissues, which is famously hard to evaluate in people.

For fulfillment, we present information on the overall impacts of IER, IF, and CER on flowing aggregate and bioavailable IGF-I. We announced no adjustment of flowing complete IGF-I focuses alongside weight reduction with IER or CER in both of our examinations. IER and CER both expanded IGFBP-1 (26% and 28%, separately) and IGFBP-2 (22% and 36%, individually), yet didn't change serum bioavailable IGF-I when estimated after feed days. There was a further intense 17% increment in IGFBP-2 on the morning after the 2 limited days of a 70% ER, yet no quantifiable changes altogether or serum bioavailable IGF-I. It is recently revealed that 4 days of 80% ER achieved intense decreases in serum free IGF-I (surveyed with a noncompetitive immunoradiometric test) for the most part through expansions in IGFBP-2, just as expansions in the corrosive labile subunit. The general impact of IER or IF on IGF-I bioactivity across feed and quick days has not been evaluated.

Diminished insulin receptor action is viewed as significant as or more significant than IGF-I receptor action in forestalling tumors in people. Ceaseless ER and weight reduction are notable to diminish serum insulin and improve insulin affectability. A key inquiry is whether IER may prompt more noteworthy upgrades in insulin affectability than CER for an identical weight reduction or in general ER. The more prominent nadir of ER conceivable with times of IER, ordinarily 50–75% contrasted and 25% with CER, explicitly may diminish hepatic and instinctive fat stores and fat cell size, change insulin receptor partiality, and inspire hormetic impacts or more noteworthy metabolic adaptability.

Our underlying randomized preliminary looked at IER (2 successive days, 70% ER/week) to an isoenergetic CER in overweight and large sound ladies. IER prompted practically identical decreases in muscle versus fat contrasted and CER more than a half year. Be that as it may, IER prompted more prominent decreases in insulin opposition than did CER when estimated during feed days. Our subsequent investigation detailed that both an intermittent energy and sugar limitation and a less-prohibitive intermittent low-starch diet permitting not indispensable protein and MUFAs, 40 g carb/day] prompted identical fat misfortune (3.7 kg), the two of which were 1.8-overlay more prominent than that with CER. Decreases in insulin and insulin opposition happened in both IER bunches when estimated following a feed day contrasted and CER. The IER bunches encountered a further 25% decrease in insulin opposition when estimated following limited days.

Leptin and Adiponectin

Leptin and adiponectin are created by fat tissue. Expanding adiposity builds leptin and brings down adiponectin. The subsequent adiposity-related lopsidedness of leptin and adiponectin may have a job in malignant growth improvement and movement through the impacts on insulin affectability and irritation, and the immediate consequences for cell multiplication and apoptosis.

In overweight people, CER just increments adiponectin with huge decreases in weight. Our IER bunch had a non-critical expansion in adiponectin (10%, in the wake of taking care of days) in relationship with a 7% weight reduction, however there was no change with CER notwithstanding a practically identical weight reduction. Our subsequent IER study announced no change in adiponectin with IER (7% weight reduction) and CER (4% weight reduction). Ten weeks of ADER (substitute long stretches of 75% ER and not indispensable Mediterranean eating regimen) prompted a 30% increment in plasma adiponectin in hefty subjects when estimated after both confined and taking care of days, alongside a 4% weight reduction. Both of our IER contemplates detailed enormous equivalent decreases in leptin (40%) and the leptin-to-adiponectin proportion with IER and CER.

Inflammatory Markers

Weight reduction with CER lessens circling convergences of C-receptive protein (CRP) by 2–3% for each 1% weight reduction, though TNF and IL-6 are diminished by 1–2% per 1% weight reduction. Decreases in incendiary markers with IER line up with this and have all the earmarks of being equivalent with CER for a given weight reduction. Twelve weeks of ADER (substitute long stretches of 75% ER and a not obligatory Mediterranean eating regimen) decreased load by 4%, however didn't diminish CRP in large subjects. Two months of a comparative routine tried in 10 fat subjects with asthma didn't diminish CRP, yet decreased TNF by 70% during both confined and taking care of days after 8% weight reduction.

Weight and Biomarkers in Obese subjects

The restricted biomarker information show that IER and CER lead to tantamount decreases in adipokines and provocative markers, and minor changes in the IGF pivot. The more prominent detailed enhancements in insulin affectability with IER contrasted and CER have been founded on HOMA-IR which recommends more noteworthy upgrades in hepatic insulin affectability. These discoveries should be checked with the utilization of strong approaches, e.g., insulin brace or different procedures.

Studies of Intermittent Fasting in Normal Weight Humans

There are not many information, as far as anyone is concerned, on the impacts of IER and IF in a really typical weight populace. Various investigations have surveyed the impacts of IER, IF in accomplices that incorporate both overweight and ordinary weight subjects with variable outcomes on markers of digestion and disease hazard, yet, as far as anyone is concerned, none of these examinations have announced direct correlations between IER or IF and CER.

A few IF and IER examines have forced hyperphagia during not obligatory days to give confirmation of guideline of the impacts of IF or IER without a general ER. Three present moment IF examines (2–3 weeks) have surveyed the impacts of substitute days of a complete 20–36 hours quick scattered with times of hyperphagia (175–200% ordinary admission). These examinations have announced variable consequences for insulin affectability in the wake of devouring days of the routine, which was improved when estimated by scientist in ordinary weight and overweight men, however was not repeated by analyst in a populace of more slender typical weight men. Specialist announced impeded glucose take-up on the morning in the wake of fasting days in ladies yet not men. This shows some fringe insulin opposition in ladies, in all probability optional to more noteworthy transitions of FFAs in the wake of fasting days in ladies than in men. This is probably going to be a benevolent perception and a typical variation to fasting that jam slender weight.

A potential advantageous impact saw in these investigations incorporates expanded quality articulation in muscle (estimated following a devouring day). This elevates protection from oxidative pressure in creature models, albeit the job in human malignant growth isn't settled. An unfavorable impact was the inclination to diminish the quantity of mitochondria per cell in skeletal muscle when estimated subsequent to devouring long periods of intermittent fasting IF.

As of late announced the impacts of 3 weeks of an IER with substitute long periods of 75% ER blended with long periods of 175% of typical admission in ordinary weight and overweight subjects with and without a cell reinforcement supplement. Evaluations following fasting days (18 hours after the last supper) showed diminished plasma insulin. Quality articulation changes in fringe blood mononuclear cells in this examination showed a propensity for expanded articulation, however no progressions in the declaration of oxidative pressure qualities. Strangely, the helpful impacts of IER announced in this examination were repealed when IER incorporated a cancer prevention agent supplement, which recommends that ROS creation might be significant in improving insulin opposition in relationship with IER. Essentially, cell reinforcements have been appeared to dull the insulin-sharpening impacts of activity in ordinary weight people.

Different examinations have tried the impacts of IER in free-living ordinary weight and overweight people without specifying hyperphagia on feed days, consequently accomplishing a general decrease in energy admission. Tried a multi week ADER contrasted and no mediation controls in people. This IER had an in general 30% ER, which prompted decreases in weight (6%), muscle versus fat (14%), leptin (40%), and CRP (half), and expanded adiponectin. It is as of late detailed the 3 months pilot information of an IER that elaborate 5 days out of each long stretch of a low-protein ER (46–66% ER giving 0.25 grams protein/kg weight during limited days) scattered with ordinary admission for the excess 25 days of the month. The eating regimen was tried in 23 typical weight and overweight subjects. Evaluations at 3 months, required following 5 days of ordinary eating in 19 subjects who finished the investigation (82% of partner) showed unobtrusive decreases in body weight (2%), trunk fat, serum IGF-I (15%), and glucose (5.9%). These fundamental information show a potential for various arrangements for intermittent eating regimens, despite the fact that there are lacking subtleties of take-up to the investigation, adherence to IER, and admission on the non-limited days to educate the possible effective application regarding this eating design in the more extensive populace.

Consequently, momentary examinations have exhibited some potential, but not reliable advantages of IF and IER in gatherings of ordinary weight and overweight subjects, some without a general ER. One examination directed in a really typical weight bunch, be that as it may, didn't discover measurable contrasts in insulin affectability, and detailed diminished resting energy consumption and brought down skeletal muscle phosphorylation, which could reflect diminished skeletal muscle protein amalgamation. Hence, ADF can possibly decrease fit weight and lead to undesirable increases in muscle versus fat and the related impeding impacts in typical weight subjects.

Optimal Pattern of Restriction and Macronutrient Composition for Intermittent Fasting regimens

The ideal span, recurrence, and seriousness of ER needs to find some kind of harmony between being feasible and conveying valuable physiologic impacts. There are various likely stages of IER and IF that could be examined. IER is probably going to be desirable over IF regimens in people. Beside an assumed more prominent consistence, IER regimens that give 2496 kJ and 50 g protein on limited days will help keep up nitrogen equilibrium and bulk, which may not be accomplished with times of complete fasting. IER will inspire a more modest transition in FFAs and ketones than intermittent fasting IF, which has been connected to transient disabled glucose resistance with the resumption of typical taking care of. The more extended term ramifications of momentary debilitations in glucose resistance with rehashed IF every week isn't known.

A significant inquiry is whether the revealed decreased tumor rates with IER are connected to times of ER paying little mind to macronutrient admission, or whether they are explicitly connected to intermittent decreases in sugar, protein, or fat admission. Most creature investigations of IF have decreased generally speaking energy admission with equivalent decreases in all macronutrients. Conversely, the IER considers have kept up protein and fat substance and diminished energy admission through bringing down carb. Along these lines, the diminished paces of mammary, prostate, and pancreatic tumors and lymphomas with IER have happened with intermittent times of half ER and a 75% limitation in sugar. IER-took care of creatures in these investigations have had a general 10–25% ER and 35% decrease in starches contrasted and creatures devouring a not obligatory eating regimen.

Dietary protein effect tumor advancement inside various creature models. Numerous rat mammary tumor examines have detailed decreased tumor rates with ER that has been accomplished with diminished starch or fat close by kept up or expanded protein admissions. Notwithstanding, detailed a 56–70% restraint in tumor development with a 7% protein diet contrasted and an isocaloric 21% protein diet in a bosom and emasculate safe prostate malignancy model connected to diminished IGF/protein kinase pathway movement and changed epigenetic impacts. The ideal protein admission to forestall malignant growth and advance wellbeing in people needs cautious thought. On a commonsense note, consistence with the energy-confined long stretches of IER is probably going to be expanded with sufficient protein, which forestalls hyperphagia. Least protein prerequisites for wellbeing and to keep up satisfactory fit weight from the general eating regimen are assessed to be 0.8 gram acceptable quality protein, kg body weight, for ordinary weight grown-ups, with higher suggested measures of 1.2 gram protein/kg body weight for more established subjects, subjects with sarcopenia, and weight-losing subjects.

IER contemplates have suggested smart dieting and not devouring non-confined days. Commonly, IER regimens tried in overweight and fat subjects bring about a by and large 30% ER. Devouring non-confined days may balance some helpful wellbeing impacts of weight reduction with IER. For instance, a high-fat ADER (45% fat on feast days) created weight reduction that was identical to that of a low-fat ADER (25% fat on feast days; 1.5 kg contrasted and 0.6 kg, however, regardless of weight reduction, prompted an unsafe lessening in brachial corridor stream interceded expansion, which could build the danger of atherosclerosis and hypertension.

Variable Responses and Adaptations to Intermittent Fasting

A diligent perception is the enormous inconstancy of reaction to IER inside creature concentrates in hereditarily indistinguishable rodents under normalized conditions. For instance, it is accounted for that endurance in p53-lacking subject shifted somewhere in the range of 161 and 462 days in the gathering devouring feed not indispensable and somewhere in the range of 49 and 609 d in the ADF bunch. This organic variety might be connected to some extent to various epigenetic impacts between creatures, which are additionally prone to deliver variable reactions in people.

Tachyphylaxis, a diminishing accordingly, could happen with either delayed boost with CER or rehashed upgrade of IER or IF. It is discovered that decreases in IGF-I during the ER time of IER were constricted with rehashed patterns of IER. Additionally, it is accounted for a metabolic adaption to twice week after week 24 hours diets, with more prominent glucose take-up and decreases in ketone creation by week 7 of IF. Then again, in lean people, it is accounted for diminishing oxidative pressure because of rehashed times of hyperphagia and an assumed up regulation of cell reinforcement catalysts. Longer-term investigations of IER and IF would permit this issue to be analyzed.

3.6 Discussion

There are not many information, as far as anyone is concerned, that illuminate about whether IER and IF have more noteworthy anticancer impacts than an isoenergetic CER routine or without a general ER. The similar impacts of IER and CER on components connected to malignancy hazard inside creature and human examinations are summed up, just as the numerous holes in these information.

Human investigations of IER and IF for the most part have been present moment, and included little gatherings of chosen subjects. These investigations don't educate about any potential longer-term variations and consequences for illness hazard with longer-term IER or IF that may happen. Longer-term investigations of adherence to and viability and security of IER and IF are needed in corpulent, overweight, and ordinary weight subjects.

The restricted information on IER and IF show a few, however in no way, shape or form steady, useful impacts, and are at present lacking to help claims about the anticancer impacts of IER and IF. Nonetheless, the ubiquity of intermittent slimming down and some sure discoveries with IER contrasted and CER mean IER merits further examination. We need to regard the notice of scientists, who exhorted 70 years prior that "research discoveries (with IER and IF) get combined with ideas and theories to develop ideas which by pyramided reiteration become acknowledged". Great exploration contrasting IER and IF and CER are needed to find out any obvious medical advantages and anticancer impacts.

Fasting can have constructive outcomes in disease counteraction and treatment. In subject, substitute day fasting caused a significant decrease in the occurrence of lymphomas, and fasting for 1 day out of every week postponed unconstrained tumorigenesis in subject. Be that as it may, the significant decline in glucose, insulin, and IGF-1 brought about by fasting, which is joined by cell passing as well as decay in a wide scope of tissues and organs including the liver and kidneys, is trailed by a time of unusually high cell multiplication in these tissues, driven to a limited extent by the renewal of development factors during re-taking care of. When joined with cancer-causing agents during re-taking care of, this expanded proliferative action can really increment carcinogenesis or potentially precancerous injuries in tissues including liver and colon. Albeit these investigations underline the requirement for a top to bottom comprehension of its systems of activity, fasting, when applied accurately even within the sight of cancer-causing agents, is relied upon to have malignancy preventive impacts, as shown by the examinations above and by the discoveries that different patterns of PF can be just about as viable as harmful chemotherapy in the therapy of certain tumors in subject.

In the therapy of malignancy, fasting has been appeared to have more reliable and beneficial outcomes. PF for 2–3 days was appeared to shield subject from an assortment of chemotherapy sedates, an impact called differential pressure obstruction (DSR) to mirror the powerlessness of disease cells to become secured in light of the fact that oncogenes adversely control pressure opposition, and keep malignancy cells from getting ensured. PF likewise makes a significant refinement of different disease cells chemo treatment, since it encourages a limit climate in mix with the pressure conditions brought about by chemotherapy. As opposed to the secured state entered by ordinary cells during fasting, malignancy cells can't adjust, a marvel called differential pressure sharpening (DSS), in light of the thought that most changes are injurious and that the numerous transformations gathered in disease cells advance development under standard conditions however render them substantially less powerful in adjusting to outrageous conditions. In mouse models of metastatic tumors, mixes of fasting and chemotherapy that cause DSR and DSS bring about 20%–60% disease free endurance contrasted with chemotherapy or fasting alone, which are for the most part not adequate to cause any malignancy free endurance. In this way, the possibility that malignancy could be treated with long stretches of fasting alone, made mainstream many years prior, might be just mostly obvious, at any rate for some kind of diseases, however is required to be ineffectual or just halfway viable for some sorts of tumors. The viability of long haul fasting alone (fourteen days or more) in malignant growth treatment should be tried in painstakingly planned clinical preliminaries in which results, including malnourishment, cachexia, and potentially a debilitated safe framework and expanded vulnerability to specific diseases, are painstakingly observed. Paradoxically, creature information from different labs demonstrate that the blend of fasting cycles with chemotherapy is exceptionally and reliably viable in improving chemotherapeutic list and has high interpretation potential. Various progressing preliminaries ought to before long start to decide the viability of fasting in upgrading disease treatment in the center.

(A) In the two subject and people, fasting for 2 or 5 days, individually, causes a more than half abatement in IGF-I, a 30% or more reduction in glucose, and a 5–10-overlap expansion in the IGF-1 restricting protein and inhibitor IGFBP1. These and other endocrinological modifications influence the statement of many qualities in numerous cell types and the resulting decrease or stopping of development and rise in pressure opposition, which might be reliant to some degree and other pressure obstruction record factors. These intermittently outrageous conditions can advance changes, which are dependable and postpone maturing and sickness freely of calorie limitation, albeit the phone systems liable for these impacts remain ineffectively comprehended. Within the sight of chemotherapy drugs, fasting can advance the assurance of typical, yet not malignancy, cells (differential pressure opposition [DSR]), since oncogenic pathways assume focal parts in repressing pressure obstruction, and thusly, disease cells can't change to the pressure reaction mode.

(B) The limit changes brought about by fasting, and especially the exceptionally low IGF-1 and glucose levels and high IGFBP1, likewise create a tumor anticipation climate that advances malignant growth cell passing, since changed cells have gained various transformations that dynamically decline their capacity to adjust to outrageous conditions (differential pressure sharpening [DSS]).

Chapter 4. Connection between Autophagy and Intermittent Fasting in Cancer treatment

Malignancy is a main source of death around the world, and its rate is persistently expanding. Albeit anticancer treatment has improved fundamentally, it actually has restricted adequacy for tumor annihilation and is exceptionally poisonous to solid cells. In this manner, novel remedial procedures to improve chemotherapy, radiotherapy and focused on treatment are a significant objective in malignancy research. Macroautophagy (in this alluded to as autophagy) is a preserved lysosomal debasement pathway for the intracellular reusing of macromolecules and leeway of harmed organelles and misfolded proteins to guarantee cell homeostasis. Useless autophagy adds to numerous infections, including disease. Autophagy can stifle or advance tumors relying upon the formative stage and tumor type, and balancing autophagy for malignancy therapy is an intriguing remedial methodology right now under exceptional examination. Wholesome limitation is a promising convention to balance autophagy and upgrade the viability of anticancer treatments while securing typical cells. Here, the portrayal and part of autophagy in tumorigenesis will be summed up. In addition, the chance of utilizing fasting as an adjuvant treatment for malignancy treatment, just as the atomic components basic this methodology, will be introduced.

4.1 Definition and Mechanisms of Autophagy

The 2016 Nobel Prize in Physiology or Medicine was granted to Yoshinori Ohsumi for his underlying clarification of the morphological and atomic systems of autophagy during the 1990s. Autophagy is a developmentally saved lysosomal catabolic cycle by which cells debase and reuse intracellular endogenous (harmed organelles, misfolded or freak proteins and macromolecules) and exogenous (infections and microbes) parts to keep up cell homeostasis. The particularity of the freight and the conveyance course to lysosomes recognizes the three significant kinds of autophagy. Mircroautophagy includes the immediate engulfment of load in endosomal/lysosomal layer invaginations. Chaperone-intervened autophagy reuses solvent proteins with an uncovered amino corrosive theme that is perceived by the warmth stun protein; these proteins are disguised by restricting to lysosomal receptors. Macroautophagy (thus alluded to as autophagy) is the best-portrayed cycle; in this interaction, cytoplasmic constituents are inundated inside twofold film vesicles called autophagosomes, which accordingly meld with lysosomes to shape autolysosomes, where the freight are corrupted or reused. The corruption items incorporate sugars, nucleosides/nucleotides, amino acids and unsaturated fats that can be diverted to new metabolic courses for cell upkeep.

Autophagy happens at basal levels under physiological conditions and can likewise be up regulated in light of unpleasant upgrades like hypoxia, wholesome hardship, DNA harm, and cytotoxic specialists. The sub-atomic apparatus that intervenes the autophagy cycle is developmentally saved in higher eukaryotes and controlled by explicit qualities (ATG qualities), which were at first portrayed in yeast. Each stage is constrained by various protein buildings controlled by the initiation or inactivation of a few pressure responsive pathways, for example, those including mammalian objective of rapamycin, AMP-actuated protein kinase (AMPK—energy) and hypoxia-inducible variables (HIFs—stress). With respect to, the actuation of the ULK1 complex signs for autophagosome nucleation heavily influenced by the PI3K III mind boggling, whose enactment prompts PIP3 creation, which thus selects different proteins to frame the phagophore. Consequently, two ubiquitin-like formation frameworks intercede the enlistment of ATG12–ATG5 and microtubule-related protein light chain 3 (LC3) proteins to the phagophore, permitting its extension and conclusion to shape the develop autophagosome. This cycle prompts the transformation of the dissolvable protein LC3-I through formation to frame a LC3-II film related structure in the cytosol, explicitly in the inward and external layers of the autophagosome. Moreover, LC3-II can interface with connector proteins, for example, p62 (otherwise called sequestosome), which guides freight conveyance to autophagosomes for additional corruption in lysosomes, the last advance of autophagy.

All through the previous decade, autophagy has pulled in significant consideration as an expected objective of pharmacological specialists or dietary mediations that repress or enact this interaction for a few human issues, including contaminations and incendiary illnesses, neurodegeneration, metabolic and cardiovascular infections, heftiness and malignant growth.

4.2 Cancer and Autophagy

The job of autophagy in disease is perplexing, and its capacity may differ as per a few organic variables, including tumor type, movement stage and hereditary scene, alongside oncogene actuation and tumor silencer inactivation. Along these lines, autophagy can be connected either to the avoidance of tumorigenesis or to the empowering of malignancy cell variation, multiplication, endurance and metastasis. The underlying sign that autophagy could have a significant job in tumor concealment came from a few investigations investigating the fundamental autophagy quality BECN1, which encodes the Beclin-1 protein, in various cell models. It is exhibited that BECN1 was regularly monoallelically erased in ovarian, bosom and testicular malignant growth. Additionally, subject holding allelic deficiency of BECN1 had a fractional autophagy lack and were inclined to the improvement of hepatocarcinoma and lung tumors at a high level age. Nonetheless, BECN1 is found neighboring the notable tumor silencer quality BRCA1, which is normally erased in inherited bosom malignancy. These erasures are by and large broad and influence BRCA1 alongside a few different qualities, including BECN1, recommending that the cancellation of BRCA1, not the erasure of BECN1, is the driver change in bosom malignancy. Nonetheless, autophagy hindrance because of a mosaic cancellation of ATG5 actuates favorable liver tumors, exhibiting that various tissues have various reactions to autophagy weakness. Besides, the enactment of oncogenes and inactivation of tumor silencers are related with autophagy restraint and tumorigenesis. When all is said in done, concentrates from creature models note that the tumor silencer capacity of autophagy is related with cell security from oxidative pressure, DNA harm, irritation and the collection of broken organelles. Altogether, these wonders are significant components that could trigger genomic insecurities prompting tumor improvement. Notwithstanding, the deficiency of capacity of autophagy qualities has not yet been recognized and exhibited in people, raising questions about the importance of autophagy to tumor commencement in various kinds of disease. Also, the autophagic hardware is certainly not a typical objective of substantial transformations, showing that autophagy may have a key part in the endurance and movement of tumor cells.

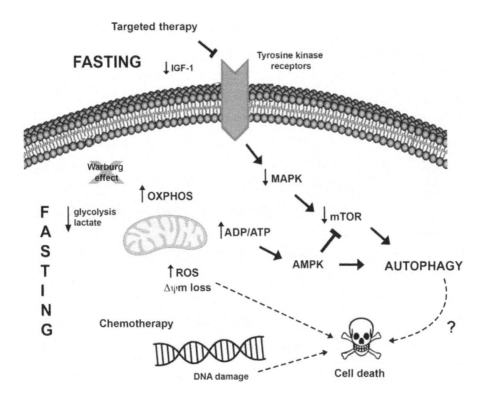

When the tumor is set up, the fundamental capacity of autophagy is to furnish a way to adapt to cell stressors, including hypoxia, nourishing and development factor hardship and harming boosts, consequently permitting tumor variation, multiplication, endurance and dispersal. Autophagy, by debasing macromolecules and inadequate organelles, supplies metabolites and up manages mitochondrial work, supporting tumor cell reasonability even in continually unpleasant conditions. Studies have exhibited that autophagy increments in hypoxic locales of strong tumors, preferring cell endurance. The restraint of autophagy prompts an extreme enlistment of cell demise in these locales. Additionally, tumors every now and again have changes or erasures in the tumor silencer protein p53, which likewise favors autophagy acceptance to reuse intracellular parts for tumor development. Albeit the basal autophagy rate is by and large low in ordinary cells under physiological conditions, a few tumors show an undeniable degree of basal autophagy, building up the prosurvival part of autophagy in malignant growth. RAS-changed malignant growth cells go through autophagy up guideline to supply metabolic necessities and keep up practical mitochondria, which thus favors tumor foundation. Autophagy additionally has a strong part in metastasis by meddling with epithelial-mesenchymal progress constituents to support tumor cell scattering. At long last, examines have shown that autophagy is regularly actuated as an endurance component against antitumor medicines, like chemotherapy, radiotherapy and focused on treatment, adding to treatment obstruction.

4.3 Cancer Therapeutics and Autophagy

Since autophagy can repress tumor advancement or favor tumor development, movement, intrusion and treatment obstruction, specialists recommended that autophagy balance could be another helpful methodology in the treatment of certain malignancies.

As of late, we distributed a survey on autophagy and malignancy, proposing that a few difficulties, for example, the deficient comprehension of the connection between autophagy, tumor obstruction, and cell demise, just as the recognizable proof of new medication peak targets, should be overwhelmed with the point of pharmacologically tweaking autophagy for disease treatment. A portion of these ideas depend on the current writing and on past investigations distributed by our gathering exhibiting that consolidating various specialists, for example, selumetinib and cytarabine with autophagy inhibitors improved the action of selumetinib and cytarabine against colorectal malignancy cells and leukemia cells, individually. Autophagy was likewise seen in melanoma cells under treatment with palladium complex medications, showing the significance of examining the connection among autophagy and apoptosis during new medication advancement. Furthermore, different investigations showed that restraining autophagy by chloroquine in mix with sorafenib in an in vitro model of glioblastoma and in mix with temozolomide in melanoma patients expanded antitumor treatment adequacy. The restraint of autophagy was likewise exhibited to potentiate the reaction to radiotherapy in ovarian and esophageal malignant growth. The adequacy of autophagy in preferring cell passing has been exhibited in numerous other malignant growth models, for example, bosom disease, leukemia, prostate malignant growth, and myeloma. Nonetheless, until this point in time, clinical preliminaries have not exhibited that autophagy hindrance related with anticancer treatment gave solid helpful advantages to patients. Right now, conventions focusing on autophagy enlistment rather than autophagy bar are under exceptional examination in oncology. In any case, no medication presently authorized by any administrative organization was produced for autophagy tweak, albeit a few endorsed specialists in fact balance autophagy somewhat.

4.4 How Intermittent Fasting modulate Autophagy and Cancer Therapy?

In preclinical examinations, dietary limitation (DR) has been appeared to broaden the life expectancy and diminish the improvement old enough related illnesses like diabetes, malignant growth, and neurodegenerative and cardiovascular infections. DR advances metabolic and cell changes in life forms from prokaryotes to people that permit variation to times of restricted supplement accessibility. The principle changes incorporate diminished blood glucose levels and development factor flagging and the enactment of stress obstruction pathways influencing cell development, energy digestion, and assurance against oxidative pressure, irritation and cell demise. Supplement starvation additionally enacts autophagy in most refined cells and organs, like the liver and muscle, as a versatile instrument to unpleasant conditions.

Studies exhibit that dietary mediations can decrease tumor occurrence and potentiate the adequacy of chemo- and radiotherapy in various tumor models, featuring dietary control as a potential extra to standard disease treatments. Among the many eating routine regimens that have been evaluated, caloric limitation (CR) and fasting are the strategies under extraordinary examination in oncology. CR is characterized as an ongoing decrease in the day by day caloric admission by 20-40% without the incurrence of ailing health and with the support of feast recurrence (68). Interestingly, fasting is portrayed by the total hardship of food however not water, with mediating times of ordinary food admission. In view of the term, fasting can be delegated (I) intermittent fasting (IF—e.g., substitute day fasting (16 hours) or 48 hours of fasting/week) or (ii) occasional fasting (PF—e.g., at least 3 days of fasting each at least fourteen days). In this article, we don't survey CR considers that have been explored somewhere else; all things being equal, we center around contemplates utilizing IF conventions as an adjuvant to malignant growth treatment in creatures and people.

As of late, concentrates in vitro and in vivo models have shown that intermittent fasting improved the chemotherapeutic reaction to doxorubicin, cyclophosphamide, gemcitabine and tyrosine kinase inhibitors in models of glioma, neuroblastoma, melanoma, fibrosarcoma and bosom malignant growth, colon disease, pancreatic malignant growth, hepatocellular disease and cellular breakdown in the lungs. Intermittent fasting IF has likewise been appeared to improve the radio affectability of glioma and bosom disease in subject. Curiously, fasting in blend with cytotoxic specialists got differential reactions in typical and malignancy cells, a marvel known as differential pressure obstruction (DSR). For DSR, ordinary cells focus on support pathways and inactivate development factor flagging when supplements are missing. Conversely, malignancy cells, because of oncogene actuation, don't hinder pressure obstruction pathways, along these lines getting powerless against cytotoxic treatment. Intermittent fasting IF, by diminishing the circling glucose levels, shielded subject from doxorubicin poisonousness and especially advanced cardio security interceded to some extent by EGFR1-subordinate transcriptional guideline of atrial natriuretic peptide and B-type natriuretic peptide in heart tissue. Intermittent fasting IF likewise worked with DNA fix initiation systems and protected little intestinal (SI) undeveloped cell reasonability too SI design and hindrance work after openness to high-portion etoposide, recommending that fasting can be applied to decrease results and harmfulness in patients going through chemotherapy.

Albeit the aftereffects of consolidating intermittent fasting IF with anticancer medications are empowering, the atomic components are not totally clear. It is shown that IF (48-hour fasting) decreased the glucose and IGF-1 levels by 60% and 70%, individually, in a bosom malignant growth creature model. In a colon disease model, IF repressed tumor development without causing perpetual weight reduction and diminished M2 polarization of tumor-related macrophages in subject. In vitro information showed autophagy acceptance and CD73 down guideline, trailed by a diminishing in extracellular adenosine and the hindrance of M2 polarization because of the inactivation.

At the point when intermittent fasting IF cycles were joined with chemotherapy, tumor development was eased back and generally endurance was delayed in bosom malignancy, melanoma and neuroblastoma creature models. The in vitro information showed that this restorative mix came about in expanded S6 kinase phosphorylation, caspase-3 cleavage and apoptosis enlistment in malignant growth cells yet not in ordinary cells. Different investigations exhibited that the blend of IF and oxaliplatin additionally diminished tumor development and glucose take-up in vivo and came about in down managed high-impact glycolysis followed by expanded oxidative phosphorylation, prompting expanded oxidative pressure, diminished ATP amalgamation and cell passing in colon malignant growth cell models. Moreover, our gathering likewise exhibited that healthful hardship upgraded the affectability of both wild sort and human melanoma cells to cisplatin treatment followed by ROS creation and mitochondrial bother prompting apoptosis without autophagy inclusion in the phone passing cycle. It is showed that intermittent fasting IF improved the chemotherapeutic reaction to oxaliplatin in murine fibrosarcoma, decreasing tumor development in immunocompetent subject. This gathering likewise showed that the weakness of tumor development was reliant upon the phone invulnerable framework just as on autophagy; IF in addition to chemotherapy couldn't impede tumor development in either subject or tumor cells after autophagy inadequacy was prompted by knockdown.

The blend of intermittent fasting IF and tyrosine kinase inhibitors advanced the supported restraint of the MAPK pathway, prompting hostile to proliferative impacts in bosom, colorectal and cellular breakdown in the lungs cell models, just as to the hindrance of tumor development in an in vivo model of cellular breakdown in the lungs. The blend of IF and the multi-tyrosine kinase inhibitor displayed an added substance impact in restraining hepatocarcinoma cell expansion and glucose take-up just as down managing the MAPK pathway and the quality articulation, which are normally modified in hepatocarcinoma cells. In pancreatic malignancy, fasting expanded the take-up of gemcitabine because of upgraded levels of its carrier, consequently potentiating cell passing. In a pancreatic disease model, fasting cycles and gemcitabine treatment initiated a decrease in tumor development of over 40%.

A little pilot study containing 10 patients determined to have bosom, prostate, esophageal or cellular breakdown in the lungs in cutting edge stages proposed that times of intermittent fasting when chemotherapy decreases oneself detailed symptoms of treatment, particularly those related with the gastrointestinal framework, just as shortcoming and weariness. Moreover, no adverse consequence on the chemotherapy reaction or diligent weight reduction was noticed. In another clinical preliminary, the mix of IF and platinum-based chemotherapy advanced pathologic complete or incomplete radiographic reactions in most of patients influenced by various stages and sorts of tumors, for example, ovarian, uterine, bosom and urothelial disease. A decrease in leukocyte DNA harm, notwithstanding diminished degrees of circling IGF-1, has additionally been accounted for. The two examinations set up the plausibility of intermittent fasting IF in people and recommended that joining intermittent fasting IF with cytotoxic specialists in the clinical setting is protected and might be all around endured by patients, albeit this routine might be mentally awkward for certain people. Presently, other clinical preliminaries including intermittent fasting IF joined with chemotherapy in malignant growth patients are in progress. The consequences of these preliminaries will be fundamental for a superior assessment of the clinical potential and use of this new restorative methodology.

Another tale pharmacological remedial technique right now being researched to treat malignant growth is the blend of caloric limitation mimetics (CRMs) with cytotoxic specialists. CRMs are intensifies that have distinctive substance constructions and copy the biochemical and utilitarian impacts of CR, for example, the enactment of AMPK and restraint prompting autophagy enlistment, the consumption of acetyl-CoA and ATP, and the diminished use of glucose, without evoking the inconvenience of CR. A few investigations showed the tumor-suppressive impacts of CRM specialists, for instance, 2-deoxy-glucose, metformin, resveratrol and regular mixtures, for example, curcumin, in mix with antitumor therapies in various disease models. The potential associations among fasting and anticancer treatment potentiation in tumor cells.

Probable sub-atomic systems actuated by fasting and anticancer therapy to advance intracellular changes and autophagy enlistment in tumor cells. I) Fasting may go against the Warburg impact (glucose breakdown by glycolysis even within the sight of oxygen), preferring oxidative phosphorylation in tumor cells and bringing about expanded ROS creation and decreased degrees of lactate and potentially ATP. The expansion in the ADP/ATP proportion can enact the AMPK pathway, prompting autophagy acceptance. Besides, the supported distressing climate can bring about cell passing acceptance. Several tumours have mutations that promote MAPK pathway hyperactivation, allowing tumour cells to develop, survive, and reproduce. Fasting and therapies that target this pathway may result in downregulation of this pathway and reduced AKT activation, resulting in autophagy induction and cell death. Fasting also enhances chemotherapy's negative effects, such as DNA damage, by activating the cell death machinery, deregulating pro- and anti-apoptotic proteins, and inducing mitochondrial alterations and caspase activation, all of which lead to apoptosis.

Impact of intermittent fasting with or without caloric limitation on prostate malignancy development and endurance in subject. Caloric limitation (CR) defers malignancy development in creatures, however interpretation to people is troublesome. We speculated intermittent fasting (i.e., intermittent limit CR), might be better endured and draw out endurance of prostate malignancy bearing subject. There were no huge contrasts in endurance among any gatherings. Be that as it may, comparative with Group 1, there were not significant patterns for improved endurance for Groups 3. Comparative with Group 1, body loads and IGF levels were altogether lower in Groups 6 and 7.

People in present day cultures ordinarily burn-through food in any event multiple times every day, while research facility creatures are taken care of not indispensable. Overconsumption of food with such eating designs regularly prompts metabolic morbidities (insulin obstruction, inordinate collection of instinctive fat, and so forth), especially when related with a stationary way of life. Since creatures, including people, advanced in conditions where food was generally scant, they built up various transformations that empowered them to work at a significant level, both genuinely and intellectually, when in a food-denied/abstained state. Intermittent fasting (IF) includes eating designs in which people go broadened time-frames (e.g., 16–48 h) with almost no energy consumption, with mediating times of typical food admission, on a repetitive premise. We utilize the term occasional fasting (PF) to allude to IF with times of fasting or fasting mirroring eats less carbs enduring from 2 to upwards of at least 21 days. In guinea pigs and subject IF and PF have significant useful consequences for various files of wellbeing and, critically, can neutralize infection measures and improve practical result in exploratory models of a wide scope old enough related issues including diabetes, cardiovascular sickness, tumors and neurological problems, for example, Alzheimer's illness Parkinson's sickness and stroke. Investigations of IF (e.g., 60% energy limitation on 2 days out of each week or each and every other day), PF (e.g., a multi-day diet giving 750–1100 kcal) and time-confined taking care of (TRF; restricting the day by day time of food admission to 8 h or less) in ordinary and overweight human subjects have shown adequacy for weight reduction and upgrades in different wellbeing pointers including insulin obstruction and decreases in hazard factors for cardiovascular sickness.

The phone and sub-atomic instruments by which IF improves wellbeing and neutralizes illness measures include enactment of versatile cell stress reaction flagging pathways that upgrade mitochondrial wellbeing, DNA fix and autophagy. PF advances undeveloped cell based recovery just as dependable metabolic impacts. Randomized controlled clinical preliminaries of IF versus PF and isoenergetic ceaseless energy limitation in human subjects will be needed to set up the adequacy of IF in improving general wellbeing, and forestalling and overseeing significant sicknesses of maturing.

Bosom malignant growth is one of in any event 13 diseases that are delicate to stoutness and the fat synthesis of the body. Greasy tissue advances the turn of events and development of bosom malignancy. In this manner, weight reduction systems that can help lower fat and advance a good arrangement among fat and muscle are important to bosom malignant growth scientists. We are likewise learning a great deal about the part of insulin and glucose in the development of bosom malignancy. It's notable that chemicals like estrogen fuel the development of malignant growth cells in almost 80% of bosom disease cases. We're discovering that insulin has a ton of interchange with chemicals like estrogen, and abundance muscle versus fat can speed up insulin creation. The reasoning for exploring intermittent fasting with regards to bosom disease is to test whether this system will diminish fat and improve insulin levels, which thus can help lower estrogen levels and moderate the development of bosom tumors.

Conclusion

Intermittent fasting, caloric limitation and ketogenic diet are successful against malignancy in creature tests while the part of intermittent fasting is dubious and still necessities investigation. More clinical examinations are required and more appropriate examples for people ought to be researched.

A twice-week after week intermittent fasting IF convention neither deferred prostate tumor development nor gave an endurance benefit to subject going through this kind of CR. This may have come about because of reformist metabolic transformation to progressive fasting scenes. CR stays a reasonable alternative as a dietary mediation in prostate disease. Notwithstanding, further examination is required with the goal that its anticancer advantages might be caught while limiting its possible results.

This exploratory investigation found not significant patterns toward improved endurance with some intermittent fasting regimens, without weight reduction. Bigger fittingly fueled investigations to recognize humble, however clinically significant contrasts are important to affirm these discoveries.

Lightning Source UK Ltd.
Milton Keynes UK
UKHW022220260521
384443UK00002B/211